The Complete Air Fryer Main & Side Dish Cooking Guide

Easy Air Fryer Main & Side Dish Recipes For Weight Loss

Ellie Sloan

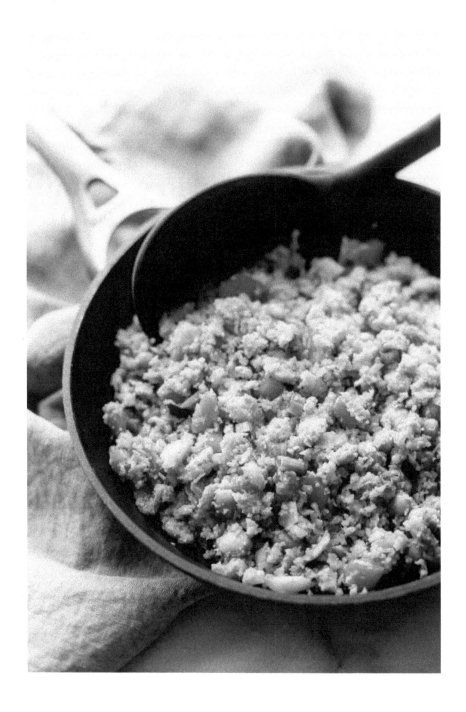

Table of contents

Cauliflower Hash

Preparation Time: 10 minutes

Cooking Time: 15 minutes

Servings: 6

Ingredients:

- 1-lb. cauliflower
- 2 eggs
- 1 tsp. salt
- ½ tsp. ground paprika
- 4 oz. turkey fillet, chopped

Directions:

1. Wash the cauliflower, chop, and set aside.
2. In a different bowl, crack the eggs and whisk well.
3. Add the salt and ground paprika; stir.
4. Place the chopped turkey in the Air Fryer basket and cook it for 4 minutes at 365°F, stirring halfway through.

5. After this, add the chopped cauliflower and stir the mixture.
6. Cook the turkey/cauliflower mixture for 6 minutes more at 370°F, stirring it halfway through.
7. Then pour in the whisked egg mixture and stir it carefully.
8. Cook the cauliflower hash for 5 minutes more at 365°F.
9. When the cauliflower hash is done, let it cool and transfer to serving bowls. Serve; enjoy.

Nutrition:

Calories 143

Fat 9.5g

Carbs 4.5g

Protein 10.4g

Asparagus with Almonds

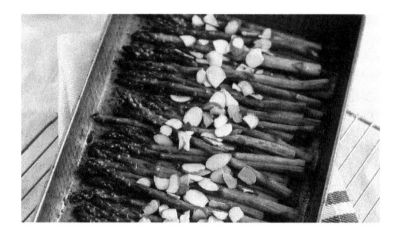

Preparation Time: 10 minutes

Cooking Time: 5 minutes

Servings: 2

Ingredients:

- 9 oz. asparagus
- 1 tsp. almond flour
- 1 tbsp. almond flakes
- ¼ tsp. salt

- 1 tsp. olive oil

Directions:

1. Combine the almond flour and almond flakes; stir the mixture well.
2. Sprinkle the asparagus with the olive oil and salt.
3. Shake it gently and coat in the almond flour mixture.
4. Place the asparagus in the Air Fryer basket and cook at 400°F for 5 minutes, stirring halfway through.
5. Then cool a little and serve.

Nutrition:

Calories 143

Fat 11g

Carbs 8.6g

Protein 6.4g

Zucchini Cubes

Preparation Time: 7 minutes

Cooking Time: 8 minutes

Servings: 2

Ingredients:

- 1 zucchini
- ½ tsp. ground black pepper
- 1 tsp. oregano
- 2 tbsp. chicken stock
- ½ tsp. coconut oil

Directions:

1. Chop the zucchini into cubes.
2. Combine the ground black pepper, and oregano; stir the mixture.
3. Sprinkle the zucchini cubes with the spice mixture and stir well.
4. After this, sprinkle the vegetables with the chicken stock.

5. Place the coconut oil in the Air Fryer basket and preheat it to 360°F for 20 seconds.
6. Then add the zucchini cubes and cook the vegetables for 8 minutes at 390°F, stirring halfway through.
7. Transfer to serving plates and enjoy!

Nutrition:

Calories 30

Fat 1.5g

Carbs 4.3g

Protein 1.4g

Sweet Potato & Onion Mix

Preparation Time: 10 minutes

Cooking Time: 15 minutes

Servings: 4

Ingredients:

- 2 sweet potatoes, peeled
- 1 red onion, peeled
- 1 white onion, peeled
- 1 tsp. olive oil
- ¼ cup almond milk

Directions:

1. Chop the sweet potatoes and the onions into cubes.
2. Sprinkle the sweet potatoes with olive oil.
3. Place the sweet potatoes in the Air Fryer basket and cook for 5 minutes at 400°F.
4. Then stir the sweet potatoes and add the chopped onions.

5. Pour in the almond milk and stir gently.

6. Cook the mix for 10 minutes more at 400°F.

7. When the mix is cooked, let it cool a little and serve.

Nutrition:

Calories 56

Fat 4.8g

Carbs 3.5g

Protein 0.6g

Spicy Eggplant Cubes

Preparation Time: 10 minutes

Cooking Time: 20 minutes

Servings: 2

Ingredients:

- 12 oz. eggplants
- ½ tsp. cayenne pepper
- ½ tsp. ground black pepper
- ½ tsp. cilantro
- ½ tsp. ground paprika

Directions:

1. Rinse the eggplants and slice them into cubes.
2. Sprinkle the eggplant cubes with the cayenne pepper and ground black pepper.
3. Add the cilantro and ground paprika.
4. Stir the mixture well and let it rest for 10 minutes.

5. After this, sprinkle the eggplants with olive oil and place in the Air Fryer basket.
6. Cook the eggplants for 20 minutes at 380°F, stirring halfway through.
7. When the eggplant cubes are done, serve them right away!

Nutrition:

Calories 67

Fat 2.8g

Carbs 10.9g

Protein 1.9g

Roasted Garlic Head

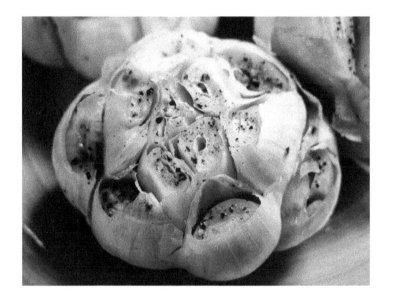

Preparation Time: 5 minutes

Cooking Time: 10 minutes

Servings: 4

Ingredients:

- 1-lb. garlic head
- 1 tbsp. olive oil

- 1 tsp. thyme

Directions:

1. Cut the ends of the garlic head and place it in the Air Fryer basket.
2. Then sprinkle the garlic head with the olive oil and thyme.
3. Cook the garlic head for 10 minutes at 400°F.
4. When the garlic head is cooked, it should be soft and aromatic.
5. Serve immediately.

Nutrition:

Calories 200

Fat 4.1g

Carbs 37.7g

Protein 7.2g

Wrapped Asparagus

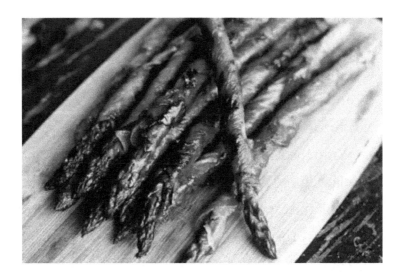

Preparation Time: 10 minutes

Cooking Time: 5 minutes

Servings: 4

Ingredients:

- 12 oz. asparagus
- ½ tsp. ground black pepper
- 3 oz. turkey fillet, sliced

- ¼ tsp. chili flakes

Directions:

1. Sprinkle the asparagus with the ground black pepper and chili flakes.
2. Stir carefully.
3. Wrap the asparagus in the sliced turkey fillet and place in the Air Fryer basket.
4. Cook the asparagus at 400°F for 5 minutes, turning halfway through cooking.
5. Let the wrapped asparagus cool for 2 minutes before serving.

Nutrition:

Calories 133

Fat 9g

Carbs 3.8g

Protein 9.8g

Baked Yams with Dill

Preparation Time: 10 minutes

Cooking Time: 8 minutes

Servings: 2

Ingredients:

- 2 yams
- 1 tbsp. fresh dill
- 1 tsp. coconut oil
- ½ tsp. minced garlic

Directions:

1. Wash the yams carefully and cut them into halves.
2. Sprinkle the yam halves with the coconut oil and then rub with the minced garlic.
3. Place the yams in the Air Fryer basket and cook for 8 minutes at 400°F.
4. After this, mash the yams gently with a fork and then sprinkle with the fresh dill.

5. Serve the yams immediately.

Nutrition:

Calories 25

Fat 2.3g

Carbs 1.2g

Protein 0.4g

Honey Onions

Preparation Time: 10 minutes

Cooking Time: 20 minutes

Servings: 2

Ingredients:

- 2 large white onions
- 1 tbsp. raw honey
- 1 tsp. water
- 1 tbsp. paprika

Directions:

1. Peel the onions and using a knife, make cuts in the shape of a cross.
2. Then combine the raw honey and water; stir.
3. Add the paprika and stir the mixture until smooth.
4. Place the onions in the Air Fryer basket and sprinkle them with the honey mixture.
5. Cook the onions for 16 minutes at 380°F.

6. When the onions are cooked, they should be soft.

7. Transfer the cooked onions to serving plates and serve.

Nutrition:

Calories 102

Fat 0.6g

Carbs 24.6g

Protein 2.2g

Delightful Roasted Garlic Slices

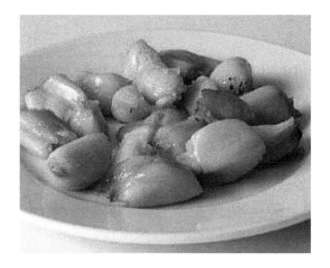

Preparation Time: 10 minutes

Cooking Time: 8 minutes

Servings: 4

Ingredients:

- 1 tsp. coconut oil
- ½ tsp. dried cilantro
- ¼ tsp. cayenne pepper

- 12 oz. garlic cloves, peeled

Directions:

1. Sprinkle the garlic cloves with the cayenne pepper and dried cilantro.
2. Mix the garlic up with the spices, and then transfer to the Air Fryer basket.
3. Add the coconut oil and cook the garlic for 8 minutes at 400°F, stirring halfway through.
4. When the garlic cloves are done, transfer them to serving plates and serve.

Nutrition:

Calories 137

Fat 1.6g

Carbs 28.2g

Protein 5.4g

Coconut Oil Artichokes

Preparation Time: 10 minutes

Cooking Time: 13 minutes

Servings: 4

Ingredients:

- 1 lb. artichokes
- 1 tbsp. coconut oil
- 1 tbsp. water
- ½ tsp. minced garlic
- ¼ tsp. cayenne pepper

Directions:

1. Trim the ends of the artichokes, sprinkle them with the water, and rub them with the minced garlic.
2. Sprinkle with the cayenne pepper and the coconut oil.
3. After this, wrap the artichokes in foil and place in the Air Fryer basket.
4. Cook for 10 minutes at 370°F.

5. Then remove the artichokes from the foil and cook them for 3 minutes more at 400°F.
6. Transfer the cooked artichokes to serving plates and allow to cool a little.
7. Serve!

Nutrition:

Calories 8
Fat 3.6g
Carbs 12.1g
Protein 3.7g

Roasted Mushrooms

Preparation Time: 10 minutes

Cooking Time: 5 minutes

Servings: 2

Ingredients:

- 12 oz. mushroom hats
- ¼ cup fresh dill, chopped
- ¼ tsp. onion, chopped
- 1 tsp. olive oil
- ¼ tsp. turmeric

Directions:

1. Combine the chopped dill and onion.
2. Add the turmeric and stir the mixture.
3. After this, add the olive oil and mix until homogenous.
4. Then fill the mushroom hats with the dill mixture and place them in the Air Fryer basket.

5. Cook the mushrooms for 5 minutes at 400°F.

6. When the vegetables are cooked, let them cool to room temperature before serving.

Nutrition:

Calories 73

Fat 3.1g

Carbs 9.2g

Protein 6.6g

Mashed Yams

Preparation Time: 10 minutes

Cooking Time: 10 minutes

Servings: 5

Ingredients:

- 1 lb. yams
- 1 tsp. olive oil
- 1 tbsp. almond milk
- ¾ tsp. salt
- 1 tsp. dried parsley

Directions:

1. Peel the yams and chop.
2. Place the chopped yams in the Air Fryer basket and sprinkle with the salt and dried parsley.
3. Add the olive oil and stir the mixture.
4. Cook the yams at 400°F for 10 minutes, stirring twice during cooking.

5. When the yams are done, blend them well with a hand blender until smooth.

6. Add the almond milk and stir carefully.

7. Serve, and enjoy!

Nutrition:

Calories 120

Fat 1.8g

Carbs 25.1g

Protein 1.4g

Cauliflower Rice

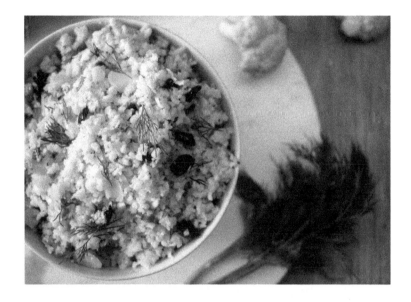

Preparation Time: 10 minutes

Cooking Time: 12 minutes

Servings: 4

Ingredients:

- 14 oz. cauliflower heads
- 1 tbsp. coconut oil

- 2 tbsp. fresh parsley, chopped

Directions:

1. Wash the cauliflower heads carefully and chop them into small pieces of rice.
2. Place the cauliflower in the Air Fryer and add coconut oil.
3. Stir carefully and cook for 10 minutes at 370°F.
4. Then add the fresh parsley and stir well.
5. Cook the cauliflower rice for 2 minutes more at 400°F.
6. After this, gently toss the cauliflower rice and serve immediately.

Nutrition:

Calories 55

Fat 3.5g

Carbs 5.4g

Protein 2g

Shredded Cabbage

Preparation Time: 15 minutes

Cooking Time: 15 minutes

Servings: 4

Ingredients:

- 15 oz. cabbage
- ¼ tsp. salt
- ¼ cup chicken stock
- ½ tsp. paprika

Directions:

1. Shred the cabbage and sprinkle it with the salt and paprika.
2. Stir the cabbage and let it sit for 10 minutes.
3. Then transfer the cabbage to the Air Fryer basket and add the chicken stock.
4. Cook the cabbage for 15 minutes at 250°F, stirring halfway through.

5. When the cabbage is soft, it is done. Serve immediately, while still hot

Nutrition:

Calories 132

Fat 2.1g

Carbs 32.1g

Protein 1.78g

Fried Leeks Recipe

Preparation Time: 5 minutes

Cooking Time: 10 minutes

Servings: 4

Ingredients:

- 4 leeks; ends cut off and halved
- 1 tbsp. butter; melted
- 1 tbsp. lemon juice
- Salt and black pepper to the taste

Directions:

1. Coat leeks with melted butter, flavor with salt and pepper, put in your Air Fryer and cook at 350°F, for 7 minutes.
2. Arrange on a platter, drizzle lemon juice all over and serve

Nutrition:

Calories 100

Fat 4g

Carbs 6g

Protein 2g

Brussels Sprouts and Tomatoes Mix Recipe

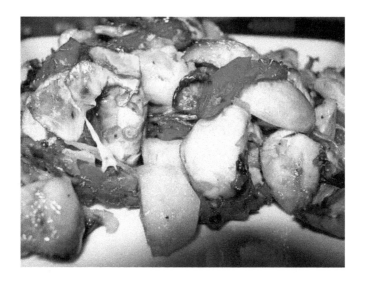

Preparation Time: 5 minutes

Cooking Time: 10 minutes

Servings: 4

Ingredients:

- 1 lb. Brussels sprouts; trimmed
- 6 cherry tomatoes; halved

- 1/4 cup green onions; chopped.
- 1 tbsp. olive oil
- Salt and black pepper to the taste

Directions:

1. Season Brussels sprouts with salt and pepper, put them in your Air Fryer and cook at 350°F, for 10 minutes
2. Transfer them to a bowl, add salt, pepper, cherry tomatoes, green onions and olive oil, toss well and serve.

Nutrition:

Calories 121

Fat 4g

Carbs 11g

Protein 4g

Radish Hash Recipe

Preparation Time: 5 minutes

Cooking Time: 15 minutes

Servings: 4

Ingredients:

- 1/2 tsp. onion powder
- 1/3 cup parmesan; grated
- 4 eggs
- 1 lb. radishes; sliced
- Salt and black pepper to the taste

Directions:

1. In a bowl; mix radishes with salt, pepper, onion, eggs and parmesan and stir well
2. Transfer radishes to a pan that fits your Air Fryer and cook at 350°F, for 7 minutes
3. Divide hash on plates and serve.

Nutrition:

Calories 80

Fat 5g

Carbs 5g

Protein 7g

Broccoli Salad Recipe

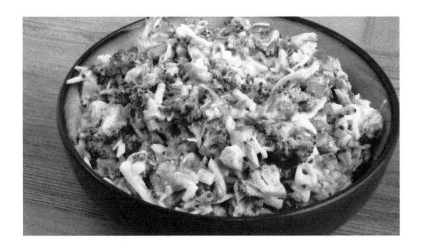

Preparation Time: 5 minutes

Cooking Time: 20 minutes

Servings: 4

Ingredients:

- 1 broccoli head; florets separated
- 1 tbsp. Chinese rice wine vinegar
- 1 tbsp. peanut oil
- 6 garlic cloves; minced

43

- Salt and black pepper to the taste

Directions:

1. In a bowl; mix broccoli with salt, pepper and half of the oil, toss, transfer to your Air Fryer and cook at 350°F, for 8 minutes; shaking the fryer halfway
2. Transfer broccoli to a salad bowl, add the rest of the peanut oil, garlic and rice vinegar, toss really well and serve.

Nutrition:

Calories 121

Fat 3g

Carbs 4g

Protein 4g

Chili Broccoli

Preparation Time: 5 minutes

Cooking Time: 15 minutes

Servings: 4

Ingredients:

- 1-lb. broccoli florets
- 2 tbsp. olive oil
- 2 tbsp. chili sauce
- Juice of 1 lime
- A pinch of salt and black pepper

Directions:

1. Combine all of the ingredients in a bowl, and toss well.
2. Put the broccoli in your Air Fryer's basket and cook at 400°F for 15 minutes.
3. Divide between plates and serve.

Nutrition:

Calories 173

Fat 6g

Carbs 6g

Protein 8g

Parmesan Broccoli and Asparagus

Preparation Time: 5 minutes

Cooking Time: 15 minutes

Servings: 4

Ingredients:

- 1 broccoli head, florets separated
- ½ lb. asparagus, trimmed
- Juice of 1 lime
- Salt and black pepper to the taste
- 2 tbsp. olive oil
- 3 tbsp. parmesan, grated

Directions:

1. In a small bowl, combine the asparagus with the broccoli and all the other ingredients except the parmesan, toss, transfer to your Air Fryer's basket and cook at 400°F for 15 minutes.

2. Divide between plates, sprinkle the parmesan on top and serve.

Nutrition:

Calories 172

Fat 5g

Carbs 4g

Protein 9g

Butter Broccoli Mix

Preparation Time: 5 minutes

Cooking Time: 15 minutes

Servings: 4

Ingredients:

- 1-lb. broccoli florets
- A pinch of salt and black pepper
- 1 tsp. sweet paprika
- ½ tbsp. butter, melted

Directions:

1. In a small bowl, combine the broccoli with the rest of the ingredients, and toss.
2. Put the broccoli in your Air Fryer's basket, cook at 350°F for 15 minutes, divide between plates and serve.

Nutrition:

Calories 130

Fat 3g

Carbs 4g

Protein 8g

Balsamic Kale

Preparation Time: 2 minutes

Cooking Time: 12 minutes

Servings: 6

Ingredients:

- 2 tbsp. olive oil
- 3 garlic cloves, minced
- 2 and ½ lb. kale leaves
- Salt and black pepper to the taste
- 2 tbsp. balsamic vinegar

Directions:

1. In a pan that fits the Air Fryer, combine all the ingredients and toss.
2. Put the pan in your Air Fryer and cook at 300°F for 12 minutes.
3. Divide between plates and serve.

Nutrition:

Calories 122

Fat 4g

Carbs 4g

Protein 5g

Kale and Olives

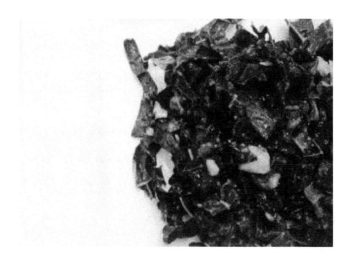

Preparation Time: 5 minutes

Cooking Time: 15 minutes

Servings: 4

Ingredients:

- 1 an ½ lb. kale, torn
- 2 tbsp. olive oil
- Salt and black pepper to the taste
- 1 tbsp. hot paprika

53

- 2 tbsp. black olives, pitted and sliced

Directions:

1. In a pan that fits the Air Fryer, combine all the ingredients and toss.
2. Put the pan in your Air Fryer, cook at 370°F for 15 minutes, divide between plates and serve.

Nutrition:

Calories 154

Fat 3g

Carbs 4g

Protein 6g

Kale and Mushrooms Mix

Preparation Time: 5 minutes

Cooking Time: 15 minutes

Servings: 4

Ingredients:

- 1 lb. brown mushrooms, sliced
- 1-lb. kale, torn
- Salt and black pepper to the taste
- 2 tbsp. olive oil
- 14 oz. coconut milk

Directions:

1. In a pot that fits your Air Fryer, mix the kale with the rest of the ingredients and toss.
2. Put the pan in the fryer, cook at 380°F for 15 minutes, divide between plates and serve.

Nutrition:

Calories 162

Fat 4g

Carbs 3g

Protein 5g

Oregano Kale

Preparation Time: 5 minutes

Cooking Time: 10 minutes

Servings: 4

Ingredients:

- 1-lb. kale, torn
- 1 tbsp. olive oil
- A pinch of salt and black pepper
- 2 tbsp. oregano, chopped

Directions:

1. In a pan that fits the Air Fryer, combine all the ingredients and toss.
2. Put the pan in the Air Fryer and cook at 380°F for 10 minutes.
3. Divide between plates and serve.

Nutrition:

Calories 140

Fat 3g

Carbs 3g

Protein 5g

Kale and Brussels Sprouts

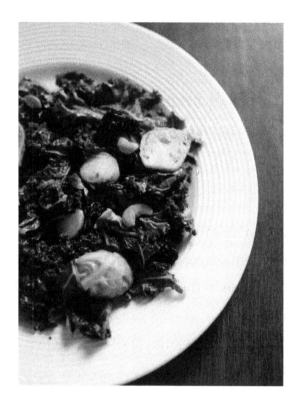

Preparation Time: 5 minutes

Cooking Time: 15 minutes

Servings: 8

Ingredients:

- 1-lb. Brussels sprouts, trimmed
- 2 cups kale, torn
- 1 tbsp. olive oil
- Salt and black pepper to the taste
- 3 oz. mozzarella, shredded

Directions:

1. In a pan that fits the Air Fryer, combine all the ingredients except the mozzarella and toss.
2. Put the pan in the Air Fryer and cook at 380°F for 15 minutes.
3. Divide between plates, sprinkle the cheese on top and serve.

Nutrition:

Calories 170

Fat 5g

Carbs 4g

Protein 7g

Spicy Olives and Avocado Mix

Preparation Time: 5 minutes

Cooking Time: 15 minutes

Servings: 4

Ingredients:

- 2 cups kalamata olives, pitted
- 2 small avocados, pitted, peeled and sliced
- ¼ cup cherry tomatoes, halved
- Juice of 1 lime
- 1 tbsp. coconut oil, melted

Directions:

1. In a pan that fits the Air Fryer, combine the olives with the other ingredients, toss, put the pan in your Air Fryer and cook at 370°F for 15 minutes.
2. Divide the mix between plates and serve.

Nutrition:

Calories 153

Fat 3g

Carbs 4g

Protein 6g

Olives, Green beans and Bacon

Preparation Time: 5 minutes

Cooking Time: 15 minutes

Servings: 4

Ingredients:

- ½ lb. green beans, trimmed and halved
- 1 cup black olives, pitted and halved
- ¼ cup bacon, cooked and crumbled
- 1 tbsp. olive oil
- ¼ cup tomato sauce

Directions:

1. In a pan that fits the Air Fryer, combine all the ingredients, toss, put the pan in the Air Fryer and cook at 380°F for 15 minutes.
2. Divide between plates and serve.

Nutrition:

Calories 160

Fat 4g

Carbs 5g

Protein 4g

Cajun Olives and Peppers

Preparation Time: 4 minutes

Cooking Time: 12 minutes

Servings: 4

Ingredients:

- 1 tbsp. olive oil
- ½ lb. mixed bell peppers, sliced
- 1 cup black olives, pitted and halved
- ½ tbsp. Cajun seasoning

Directions:

1. In a pan that fits the Air Fryer, combine all the ingredients.
2. Put the pan it in your Air Fryer and cook at 390°F for 12 minutes.
3. Divide the mix between plates and serve.

Nutrition:

Calories 151

Fat 3g

Carbs 4g

Protein 5g

Crisp Kale

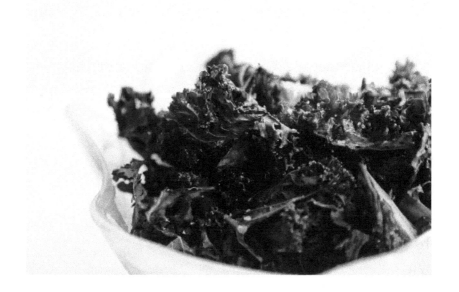

Preparation Time: 5 Minutes

Cooking Time: 8 Minutes

Ingredients:

- 4 Handfuls Kale, Washed & Stemless
- 1 Tbsp. Olive Oil
- Pinch Sea Salt

Directions:

1. Start by heating it to 360°F, and then combine your ingredients together making sure your kale is coated evenly.
2. Place the kale in your fryer and cook for eight minutes.

Nutrition:

Calories 121

Fat 4g

Carbs 5g

Protein 8g

Simple Basil Potatoes

Preparation Time: 15 Minutes

Cooking Time: 40 Minutes

Ingredients:

- 18 Medium Potatoes
- 5 Tbsp. Olive Oil
- 4 Tsp.s Basil, Dried
- 1 ½ Tsp.s Garlic Powder
- Salt & Pepper to Taste
- Oz. Butter

Directions:

1. Turn on your Air Fryer to 390°F.
2. Cut your potatoes lengthwise, and make sure to cut them thin.
3. Lightly coat your potatoes with both your butter and oil.
4. Add in salt and pepper, and then cook for 40 minutes.

Nutrition:

Calories 140

Fat 5g

Carbs 8g

Protein 9g

Sweet Potato Fries

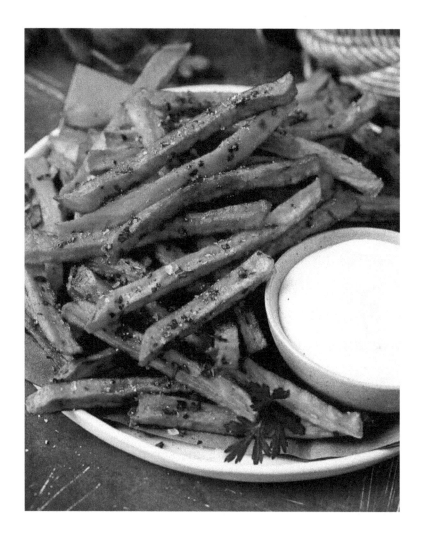

Preparation Time: 10 Minutes

Cooking Time: 12-15 Minutes

Ingredients:

- 3 Large Sweet Potatoes, Peeled
- 1 Tbsp. Olive Oil
- A Pinch Tsp. Sea Salt

Directions:

1. Turn on your Air Fryer to 390°F.
2. Start by cutting your sweet potatoes in quarters, cutting them lengthwise to make fries.
3. Combine the uncooked fries with a tbsp. of sea salt and olive oil. Make sure all of your fries are coated well.
4. Place your sweet potato pieces in your basket, cooking for 12 minutes.
5. Cook for two to three minutes more if you want it to be crispier.
6. Add more salt to taste, and serve when cooled.

Nutrition:

Calories 150

Fat 6g

Carbs 8g

Protein 9g

Crisp & Spicy Cabbage

Preparation Time: 5 Minutes

Cooking Time: 10 Minutes

Ingredients:

- 1/2 Head White Cabbage, Chopped & Washed
- 1 Tbsp. Coconut Oil, Melted
- ¼ Tsp. Cayenne Pepper
- ¼ Tsp. Chili Powder
- ¼ Tsp. Garlic Powder

Directions:

1. Turn on your Air Fryer to 390°F.
2. Mix your cabbage, spices and coconut oil together in a bowl, making sure your cabbage is coated well.
3. Place it in the fryer and cook for ten minutes.

Nutrition:

Calories 100

Fat 2g

Carbs 3g

Protein 5g

Rosemary Potatoes

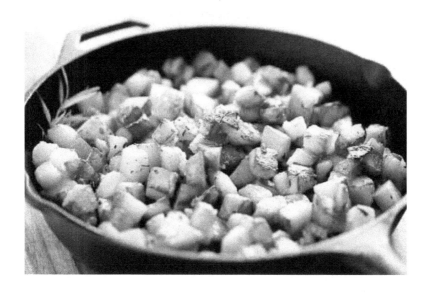

Preparation Time: 5 Minutes

Cooking Time: 12-15 Minutes

Ingredients:

- Three Large Red Potatoes, Cubed & Not Peeled
- 1 Tbsp. of Olive Oil
- Pinch Sea Salt
- ½ Tsp. Rosemary, Dried

Directions:

1. Start by preheating your fryer to 390°F.
2. Combine your potatoes with olive oil, salt and rosemary. Make sure your potatoes are coated properly.
3. Cook for 12 minutes, and then check them. If you'd like them to be crispier than you can cook them for another two to three minutes.
4. You can serve them on their own or with sour cream.

Nutrition:

Calories 150

Fat 5g

Carbs 9g

Protein 9g

Simple Garlic Potatoes

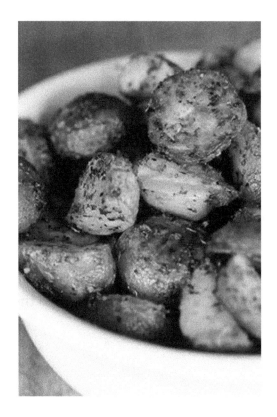

Preparation Time: 10 Minutes

Cooking Time: 15 Minutes

Ingredients:

- 3 Baking Potatoes, Large

- 2 Tbsp. Olive Oil
- 2 Tbsp. Garlic, Minced
- 1 Tbsp. Salt
- ½ Tbsp. Onion Powder

Directions:

1. Turn on your Air Fryer to 390°F.
2. Create holes in your potato, and then sprinkle it with oil and salt.
3. Mix your garlic and onion powder together, and then rub it on the potatoes evenly.
4. Put it into your Air Fryer basket, and then bake for thirty-five to forty minutes.

Nutrition:

Calories 160

Fat 6g

Carbs 9g

Protein 9g

Crispy Brussels Sprouts

Preparation Time: 5 minutes

Cooking Time: 10 minutes

Servings: 2

Ingredients:

- ½ lb. brussels sprouts, cut in half
- ½ tbsp. oil
- ½ tbsp. unsalted butter, melted

Directions:

1. Rub sprouts with oil.
2. Place into the Air Fryer basket. Cook at 400°F for 10 minutes. Stir once at the halfway mark.
3. Remove the Air Fryer basket and drizzle with melted butter. Serve.

Nutrition:

Calories 90

Fat 6.1g

Carb: 4g

Protein 2.9g

Flatbread

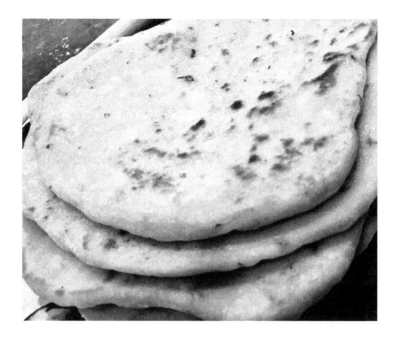

Preparation Time: 5 minutes

Cooking Time: 7 minutes

Servings: 2

Ingredients:

- 1 cup shredded mozzarella cheese

- ¼ cup almond flour
- 1 oz. full-fat cream cheese softened

Directions:

1. Melt mozzarella in the microwave for 30 seconds. Stir in almond flour until smooth.
2. Add cream cheese. Continue mixing until dough forms. Knead with wet hands if necessary.
3. Divide the dough into two pieces and roll out to ¼-inch thickness between two pieces of parchment.
4. Cover the Air Fryer basket with parchment and place the flatbreads into the Air Fryer basket. Work in batches if necessary.
5. Cook at 320°F for 7 minutes. Flip once at the halfway mark.
6. Serve.

Nutrition:

Calories 296

Fat 22.6g,

Carb: 3.3g

Protein 16.3g

Creamy Cabbage

Preparation Time: 10 minutes

Cooking Time: 20 minutes

Servings: 2

Ingredients:

- ½ green cabbage head, chopped
- ½ yellow onion, chopped
- Salt and black pepper, to taste
- ½ cup whipped cream
- 1 tbsp. cornstarch

Directions:

1. Put cabbage and onion in the Air Fryer.
2. In a bowl, mix cornstarch with cream, salt, and pepper. Stir and pour over cabbage.
3. Toss and cook at 400°F for 20 minutes.
4. Serve.

Nutrition:

Calories 208

Fat 10g

Carb: 16g

Protein 5g

Vegetable Egg Rolls

Preparation Time: 15 minutes

Cooking Time: 10 minutes

Servings: 8

Ingredients:

- ½ cup chopped mushrooms
- ½ cup grated carrots
- ½ cup chopped zucchini
- green onions, chopped
- tbsp. low-sodium soy sauce
- egg roll wrappers
- 1 tbsp. cornstarch
- 1 egg, beaten

Directions:

1. In a medium bowl, combine the mushrooms, carrots, zucchini, green onions, and soy sauce, and stir together.

2. Place the egg roll wrappers on a work surface. Top each with about 3 tbsp. of the vegetable mixture.

3. In a small bowl, combine the cornstarch and egg and mix well. Brush some of this mixture on the edges of the egg roll wrappers. Roll up the wrappers, enclosing the vegetable filling. Brush some of the egg mixture on the outside of the egg rolls to seal.

4. Air fry at 380°F for 7 to 10 minutes or until the egg rolls are brown and crunchy.

Nutrition:

Calories 112

Fat 1g

Carbs 21g

Protein 4g

Veggies on Toast

Preparation Time: 12 minutes

Cooking Time: 11 minutes

Servings: 4

Ingredients:

- 1 red bell pepper, cut into ½-inch strips
- 1 cup sliced button or cremini mushrooms
- 1 small yellow squash, sliced
- green onions, cut into ½-inch slices
- Extra light olive oil for misting
- to 6 pieces sliced French or Italian bread
- tbsp. softened butter
- ½ cup soft goat cheese

Directions:

1. Combine the red pepper, mushrooms, squash, and green onions in the Air Fryer and mist with oil. Roast at 375°F

for 7 to 9 minutes or until the vegetables are tender, shaking the basket once during cooking time.

2. Remove the vegetables from the basket and set aside.

3. Spread the bread with butter and place in the Air Fryer, butter-side up. Toast for 2 to 4 minutes or until golden brown.

4. Spread the goat cheese on the toasted bread and top with the vegetables; serve warm.

5. Variation tip: To add even more flavor, drizzle the finished toasts with extra-virgin olive oil and balsamic vinegar.

Nutrition:

Calories 162

Fat 11g

Carbs 9g

Protein 7g

Jumbo Stuffed Mushrooms

Preparation Time: 10 minutes

Cooking Time: 20 minutes

Servings: 4

Ingredients:

- Jumbo portobello mushrooms
- 1 tbsp. olive oil
- ¼ cup ricotta cheese
- tbsp. Parmesan cheese, divided
- 1 cup frozen chopped spinach, thawed and drained
- ⅓ cup bread crumbs
- ¼ tsp. minced fresh rosemary

Directions:

1. Wipe the mushrooms with a damp cloth. Remove the stems and discard. Using a spoon, gently scrape out most of the gills.

2. Rub the mushrooms with the olive oil. Put in the Air Fryer basket, hollow side up, and bake for 3 minutes. Carefully remove the mushroom caps, because they will contain liquid. Drain the liquid out of the caps.

3. In a medium bowl, combine the ricotta, 3 tbsp. of Parmesan cheese, spinach, bread crumbs, and rosemary, and mix well.

4. Stuff this mixture into the drained mushroom caps. Sprinkle with the remaining 2 tbsp. of Parmesan cheese. Put the mushroom caps back into the basket.

5. Bake at 375°F for 4 to 6 minutes or until the filling is hot and the mushroom caps are tender.

Nutrition:

Calories 117

Fat 7g

Carbs 8g

Protein 7g

Mushroom Pita Pizzas

Preparation Time: 10 minutes

Cooking Time: 5 minutes

Servings: 4

Ingredients:

- (3-inch) pitas
- 1 tbsp. olive oil
- ¾ cup pizza sauce
- 1 (4 oz.) jar sliced mushrooms, drained
- ½ tsp. dried basil
- green onions, minced
- 1 cup grated mozzarella or provolone cheese
- 1 cup sliced grape tomatoes

Directions:

1. Brush each piece of pita with oil and top with the pizza sauce.

2. Add the mushrooms and sprinke with basil and green onions.

3. Top with the grated cheese.

4. Bake 370°F for 3 to 6 minutes or until the cheese is melted and starts to brown. Top with the grape tomatoes and serve immediately.

Nutrition:

Calories 231

Fat 9g

Carbs 25g

Protein 13g

Spinach Quiche

Preparation Time: 10 minutes

Cooking Time: 20 minutes

Servings: 3

Ingredients:

- Eggs
- 1 cup frozen chopped spinach, thawed and drained
- ⅓ cup heavy cream
- Tbsp. honey mustard
- ½ cup grated Swiss or Havarti cheese
- ½ tsp. dried thyme
- Pinch of salt
- Freshly ground black pepper
- Nonstick baking spray with flour

Directions:

1. In a medium bowl, beat the eggs until blended. Stir in the spinach, cream, honey mustard, cheese, thyme, salt, and pepper.
2. Spray a 6-by-6-by-2-inch pan baking pan with nonstick spray. Pour the egg mixture into the pan.
3. Bake at 360°F for 18 to 22 minutes or until the egg mixture is puffed, light golden brown, and set.
4. Let cool for 5 minutes, then cut into wedges to serve.

Nutrition:

Calories 203

Fat 15g

Carbs 6g

Protein 11g

Yellow Squash Fritters

Preparation Time: 15 minutes

Cooking Time: 7 minutes

Servings: 4

Ingredients:

- 1 (3 oz.) package cream cheese, softened
- 1 egg, beaten
- ½ tsp. dried oregano
- Pinch of salt
- Freshly ground black pepper
- 1 medium yellow summer squash, grated
- ⅓ cup grated carrot
- ⅔ cup bread crumbs
- tbsp. olive oil

Directions:

1. In a medium bowl, combine the cream cheese, egg, oregano, and salt and pepper. Add the squash and carrot, and mix well. Stir in the breadcrumbs.
2. Form about 2 tbsp. of this mixture into a patty about ½ inch thick. Repeat with remaining mixture. Brush the fritters with olive oil.
3. Air-fry at 390°F until crisp and golden, about 7 to 9 minutes.

Nutrition:

Calories 234

Fat 17g

Carbs 16g

Protein 6g

Pesto Gnocchi

Preparation Time: 5 minutes

Cooking Time: 20 minutes

Servings: 4

Ingredients:

- 1 tbsp. olive oil
- 1 onion, finely chopped
- cloves garlic, sliced
- 1 (16 oz.) package shelf-stable gnocchi
- 1 (8 oz.) jar pesto
- ⅓ cup grated Parmesan cheese

Directions:

1. Combine the oil, onion, garlic, and gnocchi in a 6-by-6-by-2-inch pan and put into the Air Fryer.
2. Bake at 365°F for 10 minutes, then remove the pan and stir.

3. Return the pan to the Air Fryer and cook for 8 to 13 minutes or until the gnocchi are lightly browned and crisp.
4. Remove the pan from the Air Fryer. Stir in the pesto and Parmesan cheese, and serve immediately.

Nutrition:

Calories 646

Fat 32g

Carbs 69g

Protein 22g

English Muffin Tuna Sandwiches

Preparation Time: 8 minutes

Cooking Time: 5 minutes

Servings: 4

Ingredients:

- 1 (6 oz.) can chunk light tuna, drained
- ¼ cup mayonnaise
- tbsp. mustard
- 1 tbsp. lemon juice
- green onions, minced
- English muffins, split with a fork
- tbsp. softened butter
- thin slices provolone or Muenster cheese

Directions:

1. In a small bowl, combine the tuna, mayonnaise, mustard, lemon juice, and green onions.

2. Butter the cut side of the English muffins. Grill butter-side up in the Air Fryer at 375°F for 2 to 4 minutes or until light golden brown.
3. Remove the muffins from the Air Fryer basket.
4. Top each muffin with one slice of cheese and return to the Air Fryer. Grill for 2 to 4 minutes or until the cheese melts and starts to brown.
5. Remove the muffins from the Air Fryer, top with the tuna mixture, and serve.

Nutrition:

Calories 389

Fat 23g

Carbs 25g

Protein 21g

Tuna Zucchini Melts

Preparation Time: 15 minutes

Cooking Time: 10 minutes

Servings: 4

Ingredients:

- Corn tortillas
- Tbsp. softened butter
- 1 (6 oz.) can chunk light tuna, drained
- 1 cup shredded zucchini, drained by squeezing in a kitchen towel
- ⅓ cup mayonnaise
- Tbsp. mustard
- 1 cup shredded Cheddar or Colby cheese

Directions:

1. Spread the tortillas with the softened butter. Place in the Air Fryer basket and grill at 350°F for 2 to 3 minutes or

until the tortillas are crisp. Remove from basket and set aside.

2. In a medium bowl, combine the tuna, zucchini, mayonnaise, and mustard, and mix well.

3. Divide the tuna mixture among the toasted tortillas. Top each with some of the shredded cheese.

4. Grill in the Air Fryer for 2 to 4 minutes or until the tuna mixture is hot, and the cheese melts and starts to brown. Serve.

Nutrition:

Calories 428

Fat 30g

Carbs 19g

Protein 22g

Shrimp and Grilled Cheese Sandwiches

Preparation Time: 10 minutes

Cooking Time: 5 minutes

Servings: 4

Ingredients:

- 1¼ cups shredded Colby, Cheddar, or Havarti cheese
- 1 (6 oz.) can tiny shrimp, drained
- tbsp. mayonnaise
- tbsp. minced green onion
- slices whole grain or whole-wheat bread
- tbsp. softened butter

Directions:

1. In a medium bowl, combine the cheese, shrimp, mayonnaise, and green onion, and mix well.

2. Spread this mixture on two of the slices of bread. Top with the other slices of bread to make two sandwiches. Spread the sandwiches lightly with butter.

3. Grill in the Air Fryer at 380°F for 5 to 7 minutes or until the bread is browned and crisp and the cheese is melted. Cut in half and serve warm.

Nutrition:

Calories 276

Fat 14g

Carbs 16g

Protein 22g

Shrimp Croquettes

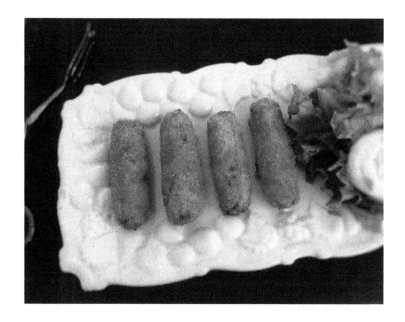

Preparation Time: 12 minutes

Cooking Time: 8 minutes

Servings: 3-4

Ingredients:

- ⅔ lb. cooked shrimp, shelled and deveined

- 1½ cups bread crumbs, divided
- 1 egg, beaten
- 1 tbsp. lemon juice
- Green onions, finely chopped
- ½ tsp. dried basil
- Pinch of salt
- Freshly ground black pepper
- 2 tbsp. olive oil

Directions:

1. Finely chop the shrimp. Take about 1 tbsp. of the finely chopped shrimp and chop it further until it's almost a paste. Set aside.
2. In a medium bowl, combine ½ cup of the bread crumbs with the egg and lemon juice. Let stand for 5 minutes.
3. Stir the shrimp, green onions, basil, salt, and pepper into the bread crumb mixture.
4. Combine the remaining 1 cup of bread crumbs with the olive oil on a shallow plate; mix well.
5. Form the shrimp mixture into 1½-inch round balls and press firmly with your hands. Roll in the bread crumb mixture to coat.

6. Air fry at 380°F the little croquettes in batches for 6 to 8 minutes or until they are brown and crisp. Serve with cocktail sauce for dipping, if desired.

Nutrition:

Calories 330

Fat 12g

Carbs 31g

Protein 24g